SUGAR BUSTERS!
Cut Sugar To Trim Fat

H. Leighton Steward

Morrison C. Bethea, M.D.

Sam S. Andrews, M.D.

Luis A. Balart, M.D.

This publication is designed to provide authoritative information in the area of diet and health but is sold with the understanding that the authors and publisher are not engaging in direct person-to-person advice. If specific medical advice is required, the services of an individual professional should be sought.

Published by Sugar Busters, LLC in the United States of America.
Sixth Printing
ISBN -0-9648149-0-0

Printed in the United States of America

Dedicated to our very enthusiastic and supportive wives: Lynda, Brenda, Linda and Muffin (whole-grain, of course).

TABLE OF CONTENTS

I
ACKNOWLEDGEMENTS

The original introduction into the advantages of a painless but beneficial way of eating came to us through Victor Rice and his wife Corinne. The inspiration for their way of eating came from Michel Montignac in *Dine Out & Lose Weight*. The evil effects of sugar had actually been described almost two decades ago by William Dufty in *Sugar Blues*. Interestingly enough, although Dufty recognized insulin as having bad effects on the body and mind, neither he nor Montignac really described why or how insulin wreaks such havoc on our bodies. Yet without their priming, what follows may have never begun.

II
FOREWORD

ugar Busters! has proven to be an effective and easy means of weight loss for me. It has changed my life and the lives of others in a way never dreamed possible.

I have, firsthandedly, observed the success stories of my friends and family, as well as my college age daughter and her friends - all of us attaining the slenderized figures we always envisioned for ourselves. At the same time, this new dietary concept has mitigated the ills of high cholesterol while improving the overall health of these *Sugar Busters!* believers. As a result, I have changed my dietary habits and feel very strongly that *Sugar Busters!'s* simple guidelines can make success attainable for almost anyone.

Sugar Busters!'s authors, three renowned physicians and a CEO with a science and research background, unequivocally endorse this revolutionary dietary concept for maintaining a healthful lifestyle. In fact, my enthusiasm for trying *Sugar Busters!* was generated by my confidence in the authors and the precise logic of their message. The authors clearly define their concept and how it is beneficial to one's waistline, cholesterol, triglycerides and general good health.

Most importantly, the authors explain why *Sugar Busters!* works and why we need to alter our conventional dietary mentalities. They not only reveal a promise of weight control but also provide the necessary facts and information that support their theory.

Sugar Busters! allows you to enjoy delicious, wholesome and satisfying meals - healthy meals that include steaks, salads with Roquefort dressing and even alcohol in moderation. For breakfast, eggs are basic, and a cheddar cheese or a crabmeat omelette with hollandaise sauce is perfectly acceptable - real music to my ears!

"Impossible," you say. "Those types of high-fat foods are unhealthy. Everyone knows that fat grams are bad." The authors of *Sugar Busters!* explain that fat is not the culprit most people think it is. Their dietary concept blames those heaping plates of low-cal, low-fat, refined pasta and all those plain baked potatoes for unwelcomed excess pounds and high cholesterol.

Sugar Busters! clarifies the function of insulin and the significant role it plays. It provides at last a new and enjoyable way of eating that can keep people healthy and slim without counting calories or fat grams.

Sugar Busters! is also the answer for someone whose lifestyle requires frequent entertaining, especially outside of the home – at parties or in restaurants. Someone who just likes to eat can be easily motivated by the variety of acceptable foods. Creativity in one's own kitchen can make dining at home a scrumptious fare as compared to the monotony of the conventional low-cal, low-fat diets that leave us less than satisfied.

The following pages are truly a feast of information for those of us who love to eat but need to lose weight — so throw away the calorie and fat gram counters. As the *Sugar Busters!* story unfolds, you will understand why.

Bon Appetit!
Ellen C. Brennan
New Orleans, LA

III
PREFACE

Why another book on dieting or how to eat? Haven't they all been written? Nearly all overlook the profound effect of one of the body's most powerful hormones - INSULIN.

Because most diets are aimed at weight loss, they have historically recommended reducing calories and/or fat; this practice is unnatural to an affluent society or even the Eskimos of North America. America is in dire need of a way of eating (and drinking) that will allow its people to consume reasonable quantities of food which can improve their daily enjoyment of life. At the same time, this new way of eating should eliminate unwanted quantities of weight and, more importantly, the adverse effects current eating habits have on blood cholesterol, triglycerides and causing, or negatively affecting, diabetes.

Is a diet really needed to enhance everybody's health and performance? A large percentage of our population is faced with the daily decisions and stress levels that were only afforded to some of the country's top leaders just a few decades back. In our lives today, at home and work and in between, we are faced with constant demands: phone calls, FAXes, computer problems and opportunities, high speed, close quarter traffic situations, and dawn-to-dawn media bombardments of local and world wide murders, pestilence, catastrophes and wars. So we all need to be ready to best handle the mental and physical demands each day presents.

Four authors? Gasp! How could it work? Well, we hope it did; you will have to be the judge. We thought it should because we are all excited and highly motivated to get a message out that should actually benefit mankind, and mankind is certainly in need of some help in the area of eating habits.

One author is a Fortune 500 CEO, sixty and slim. He has been eating the way this book recommends for over three years, is still twenty pounds down and has significantly improved blood chemistry. All this at a two year average of 3,100 calories a day!

Of our three doctor authors, we have a cardio-vascular surgeon, an endocrinologist, and a gas-troenterologist. These are not ordinary doctors:

Our heart surgeon was recently voted the number one cardiovascular surgeon in the greater New Orleans area by his peers - the most respected vote a doctor can receive.

The endocrinologist (gland doctor) is Head of the Audubon Internal Medicine Group at the largest hospital in New Orleans.

Our gastroenterologist, a member of the Center for Digestive Diseases at Tenet's Mercy+Baptist Hospital in New Orleans, is an expert in liver function and metabolism. He is extremely key in verifying the connections between various hormonal secretions and the liver where choles-terol and triglycerides are manufactured.

IV
INTRODUCTION

- ■ If you enjoy eating, this is a good news book.
- ■ If you choose to eat out frequently, or if your employment requires it, this is a good news book.
- ■ If you want your blood chemistry to improve while continuing to eat the more savory foods, this is a good news book.
- ■ If you want to lose significant quantities of weight, this is a good news book.
- ■ If you are diabetic, you can now experience a much more normal "rest of your life."

We are going to propose a way of eating that will allow you to eat most foods in normal quantities, possibly even in larger quantities than you presently consume. You can have three full meals a day and even appropriate snacks. There will not be many things you can not eat, but there will be a few combinations you should definitely avoid. What you need to avoid most will be foods or combinations of foods that require secretion of large amounts of insulin to regulate your blood sugar. By simply doing this, you can get slimmer and healthier simultaneously.

We would like to write a thick, fine print book about all this good news, but a book that covers the weight loss implications of this way of eating has already been written by Michel Montignac of France, and William Dufty has described the evil effects of sugar itself in his *Sugar Blues*.

We believe, in today's hurried and complex world, most of us actually prefer succinct and straight forward summaries of what works, what does not and why, plus a few reliable charts and graphs that prove how and why it works. We have also provided a Layman's Glossary to assist you in understanding some of the technical terms often required to properly describe various processes or facts. In addition, so as not to keep you in curious suspense for a hundred pages or more, we want to give you the essence of our findings in this introduction.

Let's get to the point. **SUGAR IS TOXIC!** Sugar? Some sugar? Most sugar? All sugar? Toxic? Well, we will say that *refined* sugar in any significant quantity is toxic to many human bodies, and it certainly helps make many bodies fat. Also, significant quantities of sugar are converted in our digestive systems from carbohydrates and starches. Certain of these foods cause a definite strain on the health of the body, probably the mind, and certainly the waistline. Sugar in fruit, fructose, will not normally hurt you, but eaten at the wrong time or in the wrong combinations can create both digestive and metabolic problems

Therefore, what we are recommending is a *low-sugar diet*. Surprisingly, that cannot be achieved by simply putting away your sugar canister.

How can sugar, something that tastes so good and has been fed so readily to most of us since childhood by our most trusted person on earth, our mother, possibly be so bad for us? Aside from a few bad direct effects, like dissolving our teeth, sugar largely acts as a stimulus in causing our pancreas gland to secrete one of the body's most powerful hormones, **INSULIN!**

Insulin has some good effects on our bodies, like regulating our blood sugar level, but the bad effects caused by the over production of this megahormone are certainly impressive and will be described at length later. Succinctly, insulin causes our bodies to store excess sugar as fat. Insulin further inhibits the mobilization of previously stored fat even if one is on a rather skimpy, but glucose generating, diet. And, most significantly, insulin signals our livers to make the other big "C" word, cholesterol.

Now you might accept the first two and say,

"Gee! That explains why I got fat or why I cannot get 'un-fat' even at a lower level of food consumption, but why should I buy this insulin-cholesterol connection?" Truth really is better than fiction, so let us relate an exchange between two of our authors.

After beginning to eat steak, lamb chops, cheese, eggs, etc. for the first time in fifteen years and seeing his cholesterol drop 21% and triglycerides by 50%, our CEO told his doctor (who also happens to be a heart surgeon) that the only thing which seemed to make sense was that insulin must be causing the liver to make cholesterol. Our doctor paused about three seconds and said, "You know, you are right! When our borderline diabetics get to where they cannot control their diabetes with pills, diet and exercise and we have to give them insulin injections, we know the first major side effect will be that their cholesterol will become quite elevated, and as the insulin shots continue, the Type

II diabetics will start getting fatty deposits all over their bodies."

Our honest and perceptive doctor immediately recognized a constantly overlooked connection between insulin and cholesterol. In addition, our endocrinologist verified that his diabetic patients have significantly higher total cholesterol than the average population.

It is 1996 and hardly anyone appreciates the insulin/cholesterol connection? Sounds crazy, but how many doctors or nutritionists have pushed that thought at you? Why have so many of our friends or patients who have gone on a low-sugar diet (not a *no* sugar diet) lowered their cholesterol by an average of 15% without either exercise or pills? How could they have increased their fat intake and seen their cholesterol, triglyceride and weight levels fall? It is the effect of lower average levels of **INSULIN** in their blood.

Carbohydrates are broken down to glucose (sugar) in our body, and the glucose raises our blood sugar. Insulin is then secreted by the pancreas to lower our blood sugar, but in the process, insulin causes the storage of fat and also increases cholesterol levels. Insulin also inhibits the mobilization of (loss of) previously stored fat. Not fancy but fact. The charts in Figure 1, page 32, will "speak to this" in a beautifully simplistic fashion.

By the way, some of us are insulin resistant and require large quantities of insulin to regulate our blood sugar levels. We have found nothing good about having high average levels of insulin in our bodies. More on this later.

Let's review the essence of our "diet" which will be covered much more thoroughly in Chapter X. There are only a few things you can not eat on this diet. They are the carbohydrates that cause an intense insulin secretion. You must virtually eliminate potatoes, corn, white rice, bread from refined flour, beets, carrots and, of course, refined sugar, corn syrup, molasses, honey, sugared colas and beer. Beyond that, you should eat fruit by itself. The list of foods allowed on the diet is extensive and will delight you by its length and variety.

Some of you will ask, "How much can I cheat on this diet?" The previous paragraph said to virtually eliminate refined sugars and certain carbohydrates. That means very little cheating. Get your sugar (glucose) through normal portions of all the acceptable carbohydrates listed in Chapter XI. Healthwise, this is the proper answer. Weightwise, some of you can cheat more than others and not gain weight, but if you have ever been significantly overweight, you had better cheat very infrequently.

Sound too simple? Well, it really is simple, but the "why" and "how" it works is somewhat more complex. When you understand the reasons this way of eating works, you will be confident it is not another gimmicky diet, and you will tend to follow its guidelines more closely and enjoy the maximum benefits. So please don't just jump to Chapter X, start the diet, and then not be able to tell anybody why you lost the weight and how you got that spring back in your step. Learn the benefits and enjoyment it can bring you for life - most probably, a longer life.

Are we the first to say certain food combinations are bad for you? No, but we think we have helped to verify why the specific way of eating we describe herein will be good for you, will help you lose weight without spending a penny on pills or spas and will have you actually enjoy eating without the accompanying guilty conscience.

Calories are not the answer to weight gain or loss. The term calorie was first used by

Lavoisier in the 1840's. Subsequently, a caloric theory developed which attempted to explain weight gain or loss. Although this theory was later proved flawed, nutritionists in the medical community ignored this correction.

We have been "hoaxed" for decades by the American nutrition industry that either did not know better or had other obvious motives. The scientific data has been available in America for years for a logical researcher to come to this same conclusion. Americans alone spend 32 billion dollars a year trying to lose weight - an incentive for some industries to ignore a way of eating that creates no profits. So get ready; you have a lot of lifelong misinformation, misconceptions and downright propaganda to overcome.

What motivates three doctors to tell you about something that will cost you only a few additional dollars each year on your grocery bill? Thank goodness doctors are in the business to save lives.

The message in this book can prolong lives and significantly improve the quality of life. The effects of a low carbohydrate (sugar) diet will actually take patients away from many doctors.

What's wrong with losing weight in other ways? Some diets lead to partial starvation, the greatest negative effects being the depletion of many of the body's essential proteins, vitamins and minerals, plus the misery one must endure being constantly deprived of normal quantities of food. Of course, a whole industry is built on providing, at a price, vitamins and supplements in any quantity you might conceivably want. Ever taste a pill you really liked? Instead of having to swallow a pill, why not eat a plateful of savory meats and vegetables and lose weight in the process?

What a waste of money to spend this 32 billion dollars a year just to try to lose weight! Why not spend just a few dollars more on your regular food budget by replacing the most notorious insulin triggering carbohydrates with other wholesome foods (foods less prone to trigger large secretions of insulin), most of which you can buy at any grocery store.

We have harped on insulin's bad effects, but we will now describe the benefits of another of the body's secretions. Glucagon, also shown on Figure 1, is released from the pancreas into the bloodstream in significant quantities following the consumption of a protein-rich meal. Glucagon promotes the mobilization of previously stored fat, so as you burn food reserves for your energy requirements between meals, high levels of glucagon will allow that energy to be derived from that spare tire around your waist. The glucagon chart also shows that once the glucagon level is raised, it will remain elevated for quite some time so you can keep on burning that mobilized fat.

Remember; insulin *inhibits* the mobilization of

previously stored fat. A high-protein meal does not require significant amounts of insulin secretion. The fat mobilization inhibitor *is not* present, but a high level of glucagon, the fat mobilizer, *is* present.

The chart also shows that carbohydrate-rich meals actually suppress glucagon secretion. So the stored fat mobilizer is absent, but the hormone to promote fat storage, insulin, is present in significant amounts. When fat gets stored, we all know where it goes!

Ready for more good news? Following the pattern of eating we recommend can greatly relieve many common stomach maladies. One author went from Rolaids or Alka Seltzer twice a week to none (zero) for thirteen months while eating steak, lamb chops, cheese and eggs for the first time in fifteen years. The only other alteration beyond a low-sugar diet was the substitution of red wine for other previously consumed spirits.

To drink or not to drink? You can find arguments both ways. But we believe, as do most American doctors, that *if* you consume alcoholic beverages, the one that benefits you the most is red wine. Populations in countries with a higher relative consumption of red wine to other spirits definitely experience a lower incidence of cardiovascular disease.

One thing is for certain: alcohol consumption does not help you lose weight. However, with reasonably comfortable adjustments in eating habits, significant quantities of weight can be lost by most people even with the continued consumption of modest amounts of alcohol like that contained in red wine.

How about exercise? Exercise is a definite plus in overall body fitness and health especially if done regularly and in moderate amounts. Never the less, a moderate amount of exercise will not significantly affect weight loss if you continue to eat foods which create a need for high levels of insulin in your bloodstream.

Our author who has lost and kept off twenty pounds is not proud of the fact that he does not take the time to exercise, but he simply does not. So the twenty pound weight loss and reduced levels of cholesterol and triglycerides did not come from exercise or a low-calorie diet.

But once again, we definitely believe exercise is good for you. In combination with the low-sugar diet we recommend, it should help with a general improvement in body weight and health.

One word of caution - if you are a marathon runner or an exercise "fanatic," this diet may not be for you. High levels of exercise require the foods that generate large quantities of glucose to feed your engine.

Does every person's body react to and process

(metabolize) the identical meal in exactly the same way? No, but understanding the messages in this book will help you understand not only why but also what you can do to positively influence your own body's reaction to various foods and combinations of food.

A few women have found it more difficult than men to lose weight on any diet. This can be explained, in part, by the fact that shortly after birth a female's metabolic rate, on an age-adjusted basis, is approximately 10% lower than that of a male's. Hormonal influences present in both premenopausal and postmenopausal women may also be responsible for their difficulties in losing weight. Hormone therapy, either in the form of birth control pills or estrogen replacement, may further aggravate this problem.

Also, please be aware that even some of the most common over-the-counter preparations can cause fluid retention, increased appetite and other changes which can lead to weight gain. However, all individuals, especially women, should be cautious about taking or discontinuing any type of medication without prior consultation with their physicians.

While we specifically address sugar's causal and/or harmful effects on problems, such as, weight gain, diabetes and cardiovascular disease, we have not stressed the many other diseases or potentially harmful mental conditions influenced by consumption of large amounts of sugar. As we and others continue to cause or follow controlled research on sugar, other definitive observations will be forthcoming. But suffice it to say, with only the very harmful effects of overconsumption of sugar that we have documented in this book, it is likely that the list of sugar- induced problems will grow considerably.

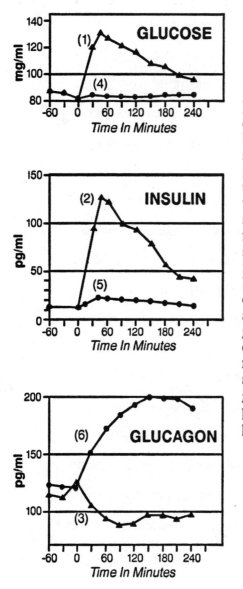

▲ High Carbohydrate Meal

● High Protein Meal

Following a high carbohydrate meal, glucose levels rise rapidly (1) stimulating the release of insulin (2) which promotes utilization of glucose but which also signals the body to store fat and prevent the mobilization of previously stored fat. Glucagon secretion is suppressed by high glucose level (3). A high protein meal, on the other hand, causes only an imperceptible rise in blood glucose (4) and, consequently, a very small rise in insulin (5) but a significant increase in glucagon level (6). Glucagon promotes the mobilization of previously stored fat.

Modified from:
    Textbook of Endocrinology
    Drs. Wilson and Foster
    Eighth Edition - 1992

Figure 1

V
A BRIEF HISTORY OF REFINED SUGAR

Your ancestors did not do it and neither did their dogs! In all the eons while our digestive systems were evolving, the world simply did not have refined sugar. A little honey for a few, yes. A little chew of the fibrous sugar cane for a few, yes. But for most of the world's inhabitants, no concentrated sugar at all — not in all those hundreds of thousands or millions of years.

Neither did those inhabitants have the luxury of being able to eat a combination of various classifications of food. They ate like all animals eat today (unless we force our pets to eat otherwise) - only one thing at a time and that was in a completely unrefined form. They did not consume huge quantities of the types of hybridized or refined carbohydrates that would require large amounts of insulin secretion.

The pancreas gland was probably not called upon to secrete as much insulin in *one day* of their *entire lifetime* as it is called upon to secrete in *every day* of our post infant lifetime! For a visual example of how we have come from zero refined sugar intake in just the last thirteen centuries to our average daily consumption of refined sugar alone, see Figure 2, page 43. And you are right; just think of how much more glucose (sugar) is generated with the carbohydrate and starch combinations of our "balanced American diet" that does not ever get picked up in the comparative statistics!

We have only had refined sugar for a mere blink of time in man's digestive evolution; think about it. Is it any wonder that the incidence of diabetes and hyperglycemia (pre diabetes) continues to get higher and higher? Maybe we simply wear out our pancreases.

Where did the observations on sugar's ill effects originate? Since refined sugar did not exist anywhere in the world until around 700 A.D., it must have been after that. The old holy books of the world's leading religions do not even mention it. Honey, yes; sugar, no. The early writers and historians did not have a word for it. If they had, they surely would have mentioned it prominently since every society introduced to refined sugar has been immediately hooked on its delights and, unfortunately, also on its ill effects.

In more recent times, a physician in the 17th century, Dr. Thomas Willis, wrote of his observation on diabetes and on some of the negative effects of sugar. Others wrote sparingly about it, or if they did write more, their works are not easily accessible.

In the early twentieth century, more attempts were made, with little effect, at alerting the world to the dangers of this refined substance.

About two decades ago, William Dufty wrote his *Sugar Blues,* which he said was inspired by the late famous actress, Gloria Swanson, who recognized sugar's poisonous effects on both her mind and body.

Dufty's research, which summarized the observations of the earlier writers on sugar, pointed out sugar's profound negative effect on early armies, even entire nations, as it was introduced to them one by one. His research makes a strong (and logical) case that diabetes and other diseases grew significantly as refined sugar consumption increased.

Why haven't the early physicians' and anti-sugar crusaders' insights or observations caught on? The refined sugar lobby has been very powerful for a couple of centuries. The economic stakes in the sugar trade between nations were extremely high. Slavery even flourished because of it. Pro-sugar lobbying by sugar growers, cola manufacturers and the packaged-food industry has been very effective in influencing our government. What politician wants to tell his constituents they should no longer eat sugar?

Is it wrong to lobby *for* one's own product? No, but it is wrong to *minimize* the serious side effects of refined sugar consumption which causes a higher incidence of a very, very bad disease like diabetes with all of its horrible effects on many organs of our bodies.

The main problem in society's ignorance of sugar's evil effects probably lies with our tendency to ignore what we do not want to hear. There have been enough earlier crusaders for the sugar message to have caught on and been spread by the most effective form of communication, namely, "word of mouth." It did not catch on, so we simply must not have wanted to hear the message.

Like an alcoholic hooked on alcohol, we are hooked on sugar. We have said, "Just don't tell me that sugar is bad, too!"

If you are not in the mental frame of mind to give up most of your sugar consumption to improve your weight and health, a half-hearted effort, accompanied by constant cheating, will not allow this "diet" to work for you. Also, don't go overboard on adding extra helpings of the foods that you are allowed to eat!

There is some interesting information on average life span that might surprise you. The statistic that man's life expectancy has increased by fifty percent in the last century is accurate, but it is nearly all due to a tremendous decrease in infant and early childhood mortality. Middle-aged American men (+/- 50 years old) only live 18 months longer than in 1900 despite the availability of flu shots, penicillin for pneumonia, antibiotics and general surgical technology including early detection technology, transplant capability and multiple life-support systems.

We also have refrigeration and improved packaging technology which allows us to eat a great variety of foods and minerals all year. And you can't go into any food store or drug store without finding shelves and shelves of vitamins, minerals and other supplements.

Why doesn't all this preventive medicine, year round "balanced" diet availability and life-support technology (that truly adds several years to many peoples'lives) result in more than an 18 month extension to a middle-aged man's life expectancy?

We believe the main culprit is the major change to refined foods and especially refined sugar. This has done to our entire population exactly what it did to the royalty of the last few centuries. Refined breads for the privileged, instead of raw or whole-grain breads, and consumption of large quantities of sugar and honey rapidly took their toll on the royalty by making them fat, giving them gout and apparently diabetes.

Just because we have everything in the world to eat doesn't mean we really eat better or even as well as most of our forefathers who ate in the fashion for which their digestive systems were designed. In fact, we believe middle-aged man's life expectancy has deteriorated - save and except for the medical wonders -and that his quality of life in his later years has also diminished on the average. Miraculous medical advances have been offset by the tremendous rise in sugar intake as shown on Figure 2, page 43.

It is quite logical that we should have added refined sugar to the priority list of things that are, or may be, "Hazardous To Your Health" when you see the increase in disease caused by our huge consumption of refined sugar and certain other carbohydrates. Sugar just may be the number one culprit in lowering the quality of life and in causing premature death. There is certainly enough evidence to bring us to that conclusion.

If the "sugar causes disease" message has not caught on yet, why do we think another book about it is worth the effort? Excess insulin is killing people prematurely, and even those who survive to an older age often have a greatly reduced quality of life. The importance of insulin has been ignored by the vast majority of nutritional and dietetic literature. The "insulin connection" needs to be understood and must be told over and over until it is appreciated.

You are the one to benefit from a low- sugar diet. One of the good old cliches is very applicable here - "Today is the first day of the rest of your life." Think about it.

Finally, the basic principles outlined in *Sugar*

Busters! have been "field tested" by the human digestive system throughout the eons, unlike the new diet claims, health claims, and vitamin and supplement claims that are long on promise but short on field testing. These new claims are all-too-often proven to be false or ineffective after a few years of research. But every time a new claim gets widely publicized, someone or some industry makes a ton of money from the sales attached to it. Following *Sugar Busters!'* principles costs nothing.

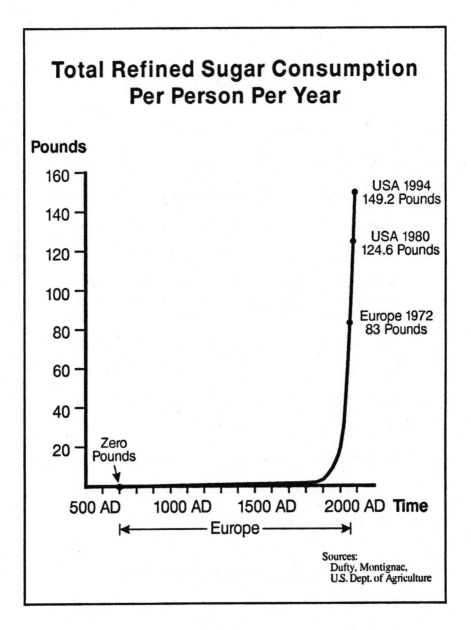

Total Refined Sugar Consumption Per Person Per Year

Figure 2

VI
MYTHS

One of the first things we would like to do is dispel some of the concepts that have been around for so long that they are almost universally believed, even by the majority of doctors. The truth is that most doctors, dietitians and other health professionals know very little about the complicated interplay of carbohydrates, fats and proteins once they enter the body. This is an area where dogma has held sway or views have been conveniently retained for many years, and only a few individuals have challenged these misconceptions. Let's examine some of these views more closely.

CALORIES AND WEIGHT LOSS

What exactly is a Calorie, and why is it so important? A Calorie is the amount of energy (heat) needed to raise 1 kilogram of water one degree centigrade (from 15° to 16°C). In other words, it is a measure of the amount of energy required to achieve a certain result. But how does this relate to the human body, and what does it mean for us?

If we were all internal combustion engines or boilers, then it would be easy to see how this concept would be important because whatever amount of fuel went into our engine would come out as approximately an equivalent amount of energy. Theoretically, if one consumed an amount of food containing a certain number of calories, the body would have to expend this energy in a given period of time to remain calorie neutral. If not, the assumption has always been that the body will convert these excess calories into stored energy (fat!) which would be released at a later date when the body would need more energy than it had consumed. This has been the standard theory for decades, and, unfortunately, it has been "scientifically" well accepted. In this mythical model, as calorie requirements are exceeded by intake, fat will undoubtedly accumulate.

Most of these premises were based on research performed decades ago - research which was not verified by other investigators or subjected to the type of scrutiny and continued refinement that is usual with most scientific research performed today. Webb tabulated a number of overeating studies and accurately determined that energy intake (calories) is not sufficient to predict weight gain or loss in any given individual. Nevertheless, the caloric theory is widely accepted and has become deeply ingrained in the public psyche.

Fortunately, individuals have not evolved like engines, and caloric requirements and consumption were never meant to be in perfect equilibrium or so finely balanced that we should be overly concerned about small variations in either direction.

In human beings, body weight is regulated by integrated and well-coordinated effects on food intake and energy expenditure, and the truth is that no one quite yet understands exactly how the body achieves this complex process. We now know that decreasing the amount of calories in the diet only leads to temporary weight loss, so there has to be a compensating process or another explanation.

Research over the last few years has shown that as we diet and lose weight, the body changes the amount of energy it expends. The body adjusts its energy requirements downward and thus needs to expend less energy to run itself (Leibel, 1995). This presents a form of resistance to maintaining a reduced weight even while maintaining exactly the same low calorie diet. This startling phenomenon accounts for the poor long-term results of most dietary treatments of obesity. We also get miserable eating less, and few of us will fight that situation for the remainder of our lives and will ultimately give in to one of life's greatest pleasures which is eating in normal quantities.

Our view is that calories per se are not as important as the types of food we eat, how we eat them, and what metabolic processes control their assimilation. What we do know is that normal, even significant, amounts of the proper types of food can be consumed for indefinite periods of time without causing weight gain!

FATS AND WEIGHT GAIN

Since fats provide more calories per gram (9) than either carbohydrates or protein (4), it has always been a popular myth that fats are "bad." This has been driven in large part by the calorie-counting myth, i.e., fat grams result in more calories than carbohydrate grams; therefore, replacing fat grams with carbohydrate grams will result in consuming fewer overall calories and therefore a healthier diet. This reasoning has given tremendous impetus to the consumption of certain types of carbohydrates, such as, pasta, potatoes and rice. This trend has now reached unprecedented proportions in this country with the "pasta craze."

The fact is that fats, in and of themselves, do not necessarily cause weight gain. Also, fats are vitally important to the body by providing essential elements, such as, fatty acids, many vitamins, and hormones which are important for the metabolic process. It is true that many of us consume more fat than we need, but this is largely due to the fact that fats are present in so many food items that have become popular in this country: fast foods like doughnuts, fried chicken, french fries, etc. Therefore, while consumption of a reasonable amount of fat is healthy, we agree it is true that it is generally necessary to trim the large amount of fats consumed in the normal American diet.

Since the ingestion of fats as well as carbohydrates may lead to changes in cholesterol, it is very important to point out that there are fats which lower cholesterol and others which raise it. For instance, monounsaturated fatty acids contained in foods, such as, olive oil, canola oil and peanut oil may, in fact, be helpful for patients with coronary artery disease or with a high risk of developing coronary disease.

Reliable studies have confirmed that low rates of coronary artery disease occur in Mediterranean countries where the population consumes a large percentage of their calories as these monounsaturated fats, primarily in the form of olive oil. Other studies show similar beneficial effects for walnuts, almonds and pecans, all rich in monounsaturated fats (O'Keefe, 1995).

On the other hand, saturated and poly-unsaturated fats are believed to lead to an increased risk for development of coronary disease. In a recent study where patients were randomly assigned to receive a Mediterranean-type diet which was high in vegetables, fresh fruit, whole grains and olive oil compared to a standard diet, there was a 79% decrease in major cardiovascular events after twenty-seven months (deLorgeril, 1993). Yet the standard diet recommended for patients with or at risk for coronary disease is to consume 80 to 85% of calories from carbohydrates with very low amounts of fat and protein! It is very possible that this may be just the wrong recommendation for many patients because such a diet can actually increase triglyceride levels and decrease HDL cholesterol (the "protective" cholesterol where the higher the HDL, the better)!

Another class of fats that may be beneficial for heart disease is the omega-3-polyunsaturated acids or fish oils. These oils decrease triglyceride levels and decrease the stickiness of platelets in the bloodstream. Elevated triglycerides, or "sticky" platelets, usually contribute to, or even cause, the start of arteriosclerosis.

Our view then is that all fats are not the same and should not be considered as having the same effect when eaten. Many, in fact, are actually good for you.

FAT CONSUMPTION AND CHOLESTEROL

A closely related myth is the cholesterol story. Cholesterol was not a major consideration until the early 1970's. At that time guidelines were first issued in the United States warning against the dangers of butter, eggs, lard and other animal fats. This produced the current trend of classifying foods as either healthy or unhealthy.

The relationship between fats (cholesterol) and heart disease was presented in the Seven Countries' Study (Skrabanek, 1995). This study recommended that fat intake be reduced to 30% of total energy intake. However, the study revealed that in the Netherlands' population, the percentage of energy derived from fat was 48%, but their life expectancy was one of the highest in Europe!

Similarly, in Crete fat consumption was 40% of total energy intake, but the incidence of heart disease was one of the lowest in Europe. These inconsistencies have never been satisfactorily explained although very high cholesterol levels (more than 300 md./dl.) are significantly related to coronary artery disease (Artaud-Wild, 1993).

Furthermore, the clinical studies directed at lowering lipids, including cholesterol, have shown no consistent decrease in death rates in spite of success in lowering cholesterol. In some studies more than half the patients with coronary disease had cholesterol levels below 200 md/dl (Anderson, 1987)! In many instances, total cholesterol is not necessarily a reliable indicator for the risk of cardiovascular disease.

ALCOHOL IS ALWAYS BAD

We all have heard over and over how fattening alcohol is, but this is only partially true. Compared to many other carbohydrates, alcohol is far less fattening. For instance, a glass of wine has less sugar than an ear of corn or a slice of white bread. The body generally utilizes the alcohol as an immediate source of energy, and while doing this, the body will not burn any energy from body reserves (fat!). The conclusion is that alcohol would prevent any weight loss. But this could be said of any carbohydrate that delivers a significant amount of energy to our bodies.

It appears that this negative effect is most pronounced when alcohol is taken on an empty stomach. Its effect is minimized if one drinks alcohol after first putting some food into the stomach, particularly foods composed of protein or lipids that do not allow the alcohol to reach the small intestine so quickly where it is then absorbed into the bloodstream.

Beer has a high content of maltose, a carbohydrate that causes a rapid increase in blood sugar and therefore insulin. This makes it a type of drink that needs to be avoided. Likewise, all after-dinner type drinks and liqueurs have a high content of sugar and should be avoided.

Wine is perhaps the most acceptable form of alcohol. It has been shown that the death rate from heart attacks is lowest in countries where wine is habitually consumed, such as, in France, Italy and Spain.

The truth is that alcohol in moderation - and particularly red wine - when taken after the ingestion of protein or lipids (like a piece of meat or cheese), will not be as harmful as one would be led to believe and can actually be beneficial in delaying the onset of or reducing the advancement of arteriosclerosis. Excessive alcohol consumption, however, usually causes harmful effects that far outweigh any of its benefits.

VII
DIGESTION AND METABOLISM

The digestion and metabolism of the foods we eat are the keys to success in maintaining good nutrition and normal body weight. Since "we are what we eat," this is an important chapter for the proper understanding of our diet concept. It will provide you with a basic understanding of these processes so that you can maximize your gains in achieving these goals. This book is being written for a broad audience (no pun intended!), including health care professionals, so we will use some technical terms from time to time. As previously mentioned, if you come to a term you do not understand, please look it up in the Layman's Glossary.

DIGESTION
Digestion encompasses the entire process from

the time food is eaten until it is finally absorbed by the intestinal cells and sent on its way to the liver for metabolism. The most important aspect of digestion is the breakdown of proteins, fats and carbohydrates into successively smaller units that can then be absorbed into the bloodstream and lymphatics to be used by the body in different ways.

Before any of this can happen, an integral part of the digestive process is the mixing and the churning (much like a concrete mixer) that occurs in the stomach. This process allows foods to be softened and mixed with fluid and be subjected to the initial phases of digestion. This mixing finally culminates in the gradual emptying of material from the stomach into the small intestine. Liquids empty from the stomach fairly quickly, within minutes, but solids empty much slower. The time that it takes for half of the stomach's solid contents to empty is somewhere between 30 to 60 minutes

Smaller solid particles empty before larger ones in a very orderly, sequential fashion. The last solids to empty are fiber or indigestible solids, such as, those found in leafy vegetables. When your mother advised, "Chew your food well," she was instinctively telling you the right thing to do since the smaller the particles, the more quickly the food would clear your stomach and, perhaps, avoid that uncomfortable feeling of fullness or the onset of indigestion.

Stomach emptying can be delayed by many external factors including the types of foods eaten. A meal containing a large amount of fat can significantly delay stomach emptying as can the drinking of large amounts of alcohol prior to, or with, the meal. Slow, or delayed, stomach emptying can then lead to the reflux of stomach contents - by this time usually very acidic - into the lower esophagus causing heart-burn, chest discomfort, fullness and even nausea and vomiting. Many of us can recall these problems after a late evening of dining and drinking and going to bed with a full stomach!

As this stomach mix is gradually emptied into the small intestine, the breakdown of foods for absorption by our bodies begins in earnest. In the first part of the small intestine, called the duodenum, bile from the gallbladder and enzymes from the pancreas mix with the stomach contents and speed the breakdown of the different foods into smaller and smaller units. This mix moves farther down the small intestine where absorption takes place by the cells lining the intestine.

It is important to point out that the mixing of certain foods can have tremendous implications later on as these smaller units become absorbed. For instance, eating foods such as string beans, asparagus and broccoli, which contain a modest amount of insoluble fiber, can positively affect the rate of digestion and absorption of carbohydrates. This causes these carbohydrates to have a much lower insulin stimulating effect. This would obviously be a good thing for the body.

Fruits eaten by themselves are also digested and absorbed at better rates than if eaten together with other carbohydrates and fats. The negative effect that eating fruits at the wrong time can have on the other foods in the digestive process is covered in Chapter XII.

METABOLISM

Metabolize essentially means "to change" and entails the many processes that transform the nutrients in food to chemical substances that can be utilized by our bodies. The entire process is obviously quite complex. The rate of, or response to, metabolism can vary considerably from person to person. This means weight gain or loss for two people on the identical diet can vary considerably.

Although the process is complex, you should know that the liver plays the central role in the metabolism of foods, including alcohol, and in the metabolism of the majority of medications. So it is easy to see the importance of the liver in our nutritional well-being, and it behooves us all to take very good care of it because medical science cannot yet duplicate its functions. When the liver goes, "Adios, Amigo!"

Now let's talk about what types of food get metabolized for use by our bodies.

PROTEINS

Proteins - the source of which are meats, nuts, dairy products, etc. - are made of subunits called amino acids. These amino acids are released from the protein by the action of enzymes secreted by the pancreas. Without these enzymes, protein molecules would not be absorbed since they are too large and complex to enter the bloodstream. Fortunately, in cases where pancreatic enzymes are missing, they can be provided in capsule form which can be taken with meals to aid the digestive process.

An average adult should consume *at least* one gram of protein for each kilogram (2.2 pounds) of weight or somewhere between 55 and 70 grams (2 to 2.5 ounces) for the average man or woman.

Since there are both animal and vegetable sources of proteins and neither of these sources provides all of the amino acids that the body needs, a diet should be well-balanced in order to provide both sources of protein.

Once proteins have been broken down into amino acids, they can be absorbed from the intestine and metabolized by the liver. Then, in general, amino acids can be either utilized by the body as the basic building blocks of all proteins, which make up all cells, hormones and neurotransmitters (substances that relay signals in the nervous system); or amino acids can be converted into glucose, or sugar, by the liver through a process called gluco-neogenesis which is the manufacture of glucose from non- carbohydrate food sources like protein.

The body's ability to manufacture its own glucose is important for the maintenance of normal energy requirements during periods of low carbohydrate consumption since glucose is the main fuel the body uses to meet its energy requirements.

CARBOHYDRATES

Carbohydrates can be found in both plant and animal food sources. The overwhelming majority of the carbohydrates we eat are in the form of starches and sugars. Carbohydrates can be classified as simple sugars or more complex sugars, such as, starch.

All carbohydrates absorbed by the body are eventually converted to glucose. Glucose is the body's main fuel, much like the gasoline that is put in a car. Glucose is either used immediately to provide energy or stored in the form of glycogen in the liver and in muscle to be utilized later.

In understanding the metabolism of carbohydrates and how this relates to our recommendations for good nutrition and weight loss, it is very important to think of carbohydrates in terms of how much of a peak or rise of glucose they can cause within the body when eaten. This can be more simply called the glycemic potential which varies for different types of carbohydrates and, in more scientific terms, can be defined as the glycemic index. The glycemic index (example shown in Figure 3, page 69) simply reflects the area under the curve representing the rise in blood sugar over a given period of time. Glucose has been assigned a relative value of 100 as its glycemic index, and the value of other carbohydrates are simply related to this level. Some substances actually have a higher glycemic potential than glucose! More on the importance of a carbohydrate's glycemic potential later.

When the blood glucose level drops lower than it should be, glycogen, which is glucose in its stored form in the body, is broken down into glucose in order to raise the level of glucose and maintain a normal blood sugar level, just as insulin comes into play to lower the glucose or blood sugar to a normal level.

Carbohydrates, such as, starches, which have a more complex structure, can, contrary to some commonly held beliefs, be digested and absorbed nearly as fast as the more simple carbohydrates, such as, table sugar. When a carbohydrate is eaten, there is a rise in the level of blood glucose commensurate with the type of carbohydrate ingested (i.e., higher for sugar, lower for fresh fruit). This rise in blood sugar (glucose) is then followed by the release of insulin which causes a fall in the level of glucose primarily as it is driven into the cells of the body where it can be utilized as instant fuel or stored mainly as fat. Following this, the glucose level returns to its normal baseline.

FATS
Fats, or lipids, are complex molecules composed of fatty acids and are derived from both animal and

vegetable origins. Fats must be digested through the actions of pancreatic enzymes called lipases; otherwise, they cannot enter the body to any great extent and are passed in the stool. Even after fats are broken down into subunits, most of these remain insoluble in water and require a special type of absorption. Bile from the liver, which is stored in the gallbladder, plays a very important role in this absorption of fats by emulsifying or dissolving them. This is akin to using soap or any detergent to help in dissolving an oily substance. Without this process, fat subunits would be too large to enter the bloodstream from the intestine.

Some individuals who lack pancreatic enzymes must take enzymes with their food. Fats are absorbed through the intestinal tract as glycerols and are reconstituted while still in the intestinal wall as triglycerides which then enter the lymphatic system where these fats can be used by all the body's cells.

Cells use fat as fuel for energy production, as an important component of cell structures and as a source of many essential substances manufactured by cells. An important function of fat that no one likes to think of is to provide insulation in the form of a layer of fat immediately underneath the skin. This should be only a thin layer, however, and it is almost always a source of constant restructuring in modern man's attempts to control weight and body shape.

Cholesterol is a unique story. Despite common belief, cholesterol is not a fat and has nothing to do with saturated fats. It is a compound belonging to a family of substances called sterols. Cholesterol can combine with fat as it circulates in the bloodstream to be distributed to all cells. Cholesterol is a vital substance in the formation of steroids, bile acids, and other substances.

Because cholesterol is so important, the body must provide a constant supply of cholesterol to the cells. Therefore, the body not only takes in cholesterol from food but also manufactures it, primarily in the liver. The liver can provide enough cholesterol to meet the body's needs even if a person were to consume no cholesterol in food!

Cholesterol manufactured in the liver circulates as lipoproteins for delivery to the cells. It is during this circulation in the bloodstream that cholesterol can be deposited on major blood vessel or artery walls, especially at points of irritation, roughness or small breaks in the lining. This is the process referred to as arteriosclerosis and is the underlying process leading to coronary heart disease and, in many cases, hypertension (high blood pressure).

Now you know how your digestive system works and some of the things that help or hinder its efficiency. We keep mentioning and hinting at the importance of insulin. The next chapter is dedicated to helping you better understand the insulin connection.

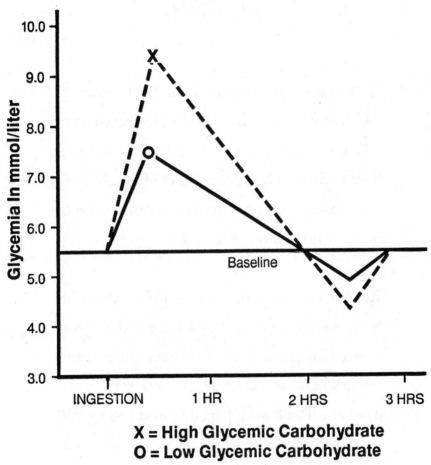

X = High Glycemic Carbohydrate
O = Low Glycemic Carbohydrate

Figure 3

VIII
INSULIN

You may ask "Why do I want to know more about insulin? It is just another seven letter hormone." Insulin is the maestro, the conductor, the chief. It is the CEO of metabolism. We must understand the actions of insulin to understand why the diet works.

Ready for some additional technical, but hopefully interesting, information? Banting and Best discovered insulin in 1921. This hormone is manufactured and secreted by the beta cells of the pancreas. The human pancreas stores about 200 units of insulin. Normal people secrete about 25-30 units of insulin daily. Insulin is like a broom. It sweeps glucose into cells where potential energy is stored as fat and glycogen to be utilized later.

In normal individuals blood-sugar levels do not

vary much. This is because of the harmonious and compensating hormone actions of insulin and glucagon. Insulin is the only hormone that can prevent sugar (glucose) from rising to dangerously high levels. Glucagon, also secreted by the pancreas, prevents the blood sugar from falling too low (to hypoglycemic levels).

Glucagon is another hormone secreted by the pancreas. Whereas insulin has been referred to as the hormone of feasting, glucagon is the hormone of fasting (or starvation). The main role of glucagon in humans appears to be the prevention of hypoglycemia (low blood glucose or blood sugar) by causing the normal breakdown of glycogen in the liver to form glucose and also gluconeogenesis which is the conversion of muscle protein to blood sugar.

Gluconeogenesis can occur during periods of starvation or excessive exercise. During the first 24 hours of fasting, glycogen in the liver is utilized and then the body will begin using up muscle proteins. So glucagon secretion is stimulated by hypoglycemia, fasting and also by the ingestion of a protein-rich meal.

Individuals can survive without glucagon as in cases where the pancreas, which is the only known source of glucagon and insulin, is removed. However, a person must have insulin to survive, and this can be accomplished through insulin injections. Of course, the result of removing the pancreas is general elevation in the blood sugar since insulin given by injections is not as efficient in providing a continuous supply in exactly the right amount as is the pancreas itself.

After a person eats carbohydrates, the digestive enzymes break down the food. The blood that is draining the intestines then picks up these simplified food substances and now, with an elevated glucose, passes by the pancreas stimulating the release of insulin. As we have previously learned, insulin causes the storage of fat. When the blood sugar falls too low, glucagon is secreted which remobilizes stored fat (yea!) into glucose which raises blood sugar back to its normal level.

Glucose is the major stimulus for insulin secretion. Fructose, a sugar from fruits, and amino acids (proteins) from meats cause a significant release of insulin only in the presence of previously elevated blood sugar. The overweight person probably has increased insulin production because of excessive stimulation of the pancreas through overeating and the development of, or genetic tendency toward, insulin resistance.

The increased insulin level promotes storage of some sugar as glycogen in the liver and the muscles. In addition, it causes storage of protein in muscles and fat in fat cells. Excess sugar is converted to and often stored as **FAT!** Insulin also prevents the breakdown of (previously stored) glycogen and triglycerides (fat). No wonder it is difficult to lose weight in the presence of elevated insulin levels.

Scientific literature documents that even low levels of circulating insulin inhibit fat breakdown (Joslin's, 1994). Higher levels are required to control blood sugars. The metabolic pathways involving insulin are exquisitely sensitive in causing the storage of fat and inhibiting its breakdown for use by the body.

Insulin further activates an enzyme, lipoprotein lipase (Enzymes are proteins that speed up metabolic actions.), that promotes the removal of triglycerides from the bloodstream and their deposition as fat cells. Insulin also inhibits hormone sensitive lipase (another enzyme) that breaks down stored fats. The net results of these two activities is an increase in stored fat which results in a weight gain.

Also adding to the fat storage is the conversion

of some of the sugar present in the blood. A percentage of the blood sugar is taken up by fat cells and, under the influence of our old friend insulin, is converted to still more fat. For our scientific readers, this involves glycerol 3-phosphate and free fatty acids. So insulin is a major deterrent to fat breakdown and a major facilitator of fat storage.

Insulin resistance is a condition of decreased responsiveness to insulin wherein the fat cells, liver cells and muscle cells have become insensitive to normal levels of circulating insulin. Usually a small burst of insulin will lower blood sugar. However, in an insulin- resistant individual, this does not occur, and more insulin is required to do the job.

Obesity is the most common result of insulin resistance. Another frequently seen result of insulin resistance is Type II diabetes. In most Type II diabetics the circulating insulin levels and

blood sugars are elevated as well as the blood cholesterol levels.

Obese individuals without diabetes usually have
elevated insulin levels with normal blood sugar levels. Unfortunately, the obese person with
an elevated insulin level may be on his way to developing diabetes. The pancreas may simply become
exhausted from constant stimulation by glucose
(sugar) and finally fail, resulting in diabetes.

Insulin promotes the storage of all foods: glucose
(carbohydrates), triglycerides (fats), and amino
acids (proteins). These stored foods are available for
use as an energy source later in a fasting state or simply between meals. The fall in insulin levels during
fasting allows the breakdown of stored fat and
stored sugar (glycogen). Fats and glycogen are then
used as energy sources between meals.

As mentioned above, obese people have elevated insulin levels in both the fasting and fed

states. Lipoprotein lipase levels are also elevated in the obese. This is the particular enzyme that is important in the storage of fat. You can now see that obese individuals are metabolically ready at all times to store whatever they eat.

Again, it's no wonder that the obese person with an elevated insulin level has a hard time losing weight. But think of the benefits of a diet for this very same person that requires the presence of very little insulin in the system. We are now gaining on the answer of how to lose weight and improve our blood chemistry at the same time.

Syndrome X, described by Dr. G.M. Reaven, is a combination of two or more of the following conditions: insulin resistance with resulting elevated insulin levels, elevated lipids (especially triglycerides), obesity, coronary artery disease, and hypertension. Insulin resistance is probably the most important part of this syndrome because, in fact, it often causes the other problems to occur. A significant number of patients with Syndrome X develop coronary artery disease and experience an increased number of fatal heart attacks (O'Keefe, 1995).

How about some good news? Fifty percent or more of insulin resistance can be reduced or even reversed since insulin resistance is not necessarily dependent on our inherited genes. How can we decrease insulin levels or reduce insulin resistance? You are right! It's the same diet or way of eating. First, we must eat less of the particularly insulin-stimulating carbohydrates. This helps with weight loss and, combined with exercise and smoking cessation, provides major non-medical ways to accomplish this reduction. So by lowering the insulin levels and decreasing insulin resistance, the incidence of obesity will decrease and probably the progression of heart disease.

Many people with coronary artery disease have similar body shapes. They are fatter in the abdomen, having beer bellies, and are thinner in the hips and buttocks. This is called central obesity (apple shape). Individuals with diabetes and insulin resistance have similar apple shapes as opposed to pear shapes where the fat is distributed in the hips and buttocks. Now we see that weight loss through a low-glycemic diet can lower insulin levels as well as triglyceride and cholesterol levels.

Dr. Wolever and coworkers in 1992 studied this type of diet in overweight non-insulin dependent diabetics. They found a 7% drop in cholesterol after only six weeks. Dr. Jenkins studied a low- glycemic (low-sugar) diet fed to normal males. After two weeks the cholesterol dropped an average of 15%, and the insulin secretion dropped an amazing 32%!

After ingestion of 50-100 grams of glucose (equal to one normally sugared soft drink) during a high-sugar meal, insulin levels usually become very elevated and can remain elevated for several hours. Eating high-carbohydrate (high-glycemic) meals three times a day and at bedtime can cause insulin to be elevated for 18 out of 24 hours. The pancreas needs a rest, and so do fat cells. Imagine insulin pushing fat into cells 18 hours a day. Only a few hours a day would be left for fat breakdown and fat loss. Fat would tend to accumulate at essentially all other times resulting in you know what going you know where!

Understanding insulin and metabolism will now enable us to follow a healthier diet. As mentioned earlier, all carbohydrates are not equal in their ability to stimulate insulin release. Carbohydrates that stimulate the most insulin secretion are called high-glycemic carbohydrates. Conversely, low-glycemic carbohydrates do not stimulate as much insulin secretion.

Since we have learned that we need to dodge the carbohydrates with the high-glycemic indexes, we are now going to provide you with some additional glycemic index information. In 1981 Dr. David Jenkins published an article on the glycemic index of foods in the *American Journal of Clinical Nutrition*. He and others have since provided many additional measurements on the glycemic indexes of certain carbohydrates.

The natural foods with the lowest glycemic indexes are beans and lentils. Lentils have an index of 29 as compared with the standard for glucose which has an index of 100. Most fruits have a low index except bananas - 60 and raisins - 65. Pumpernickel and rye breads without added forms of sugar have been studied and have an acceptable index of 45. Most other breads are best avoided because they are either made from refined flour or have had sugar added (white breads range in value from 70 to 95). Of course, stoneground, wholegrain breads without added sugar, should be "OK." Figure 4 represents the glycemic index on many commonly consumed foods.

Figure 4

GLYCEMIC INDEX

HIGH		MODERATE Cont'd.	
maltose	105	grapes	50
glucose	100	sweet potatoes	50
potatoes	70-95	wheat grains	45
white breads	95	whole grain	
parsnips	95	pasta	45
honey	90	sponge cake	45
carrots	85	pears	45
corn/cornflakes	70-85	orange juice	45
refined sugar	75	apple juice	40
millet	75	pineapple juice	40
whole wheat		oranges	40
bread	75	apples	40
beets	70	oatmeal	40
white rice	70		
refined pasta	65		
raisins	65	LOW	
plain crackers	65	milk, yogurt	35
bananas	60	dried apricots	35
		beans & peas	30-40
		peaches	30
MODERATE		plums	25
All Bran	55	fructose (alone)	20
brown rice	55	soybeans	15
whole rice	50	peanuts	10
whole grain		green vegetables	0-15
breads	40-50		

All of the above have no added sugar.
Compiled from multiple glycemic index studies.
Some numbers slightly rounded.

IX
DIET AND THE
CARDIOVASCULAR SYSTEM

Most of us follow a specific diet for one or two reasons. These are usually to enhance our appearance or improve our cardiovascular health. From an appearance point of view, being slender seems to be considered more attractive by both men and women in America today. Most of us have tried, successfully or unsuccessfully, to shed a few extra pounds before vacation or some equally important event. More recently, dieting to improve our health is gaining greater importance. The cardiovascular system is often the end point of these efforts. Therefore, we would like to elaborate a little about the importance of the cardiovascular system and the influence of diet.

Diseases of the cardiovascular system - primarily heart attack, hypertension and stroke - are public enemy number one, accounting for twelve million deaths annually. Coronary heart disease is the leading cause of death in industrialized countries, and in the next ten years, coronary artery disease and stroke will be the leading cause of death in most developing countries.

Heart disease, stroke and, frequently, hypertension are due to the deterioration of arteries through a process called atherosclerosis, arteriosclerosis, or just plain hardening of the arteries. This process is a natural phenomenon of aging. As we get older, so do our arteries. The smooth inner lining called the intima begins to crack when the middle elastic, muscular layer can no longer fully recoil after a pulse wave has expanded the vessel. In these cracks, platelets, fibrin, calcium, cholesterol and fat accumulate creating an atheroma, or plaque.

With continued stress on the arterial wall and further intimal (the innermost coat) disruption associated with turbulence of blood flow, more material is deposited until the artery is narrowed significantly, producing reduced blood flow to the corresponding area of the body. We now refer to the process as a disease; its presence has caused a problem.

A frequent question asked physicians is "How do I avoid getting arteriosclerosis?" The answer is easy. Don't live long enough. But most patients do not like this alternative. However, there are factors which predispose one to premature or early arteriosclerosis and subsequently to cardiovascular disease and which are important to be aware of and to plan for accordingly. Some we can alter. Others we cannot. But the knowledge gleaned from being aware of them is usually very helpful in assisting us to enhance cardiovascular fitness or health.

Initially, there were thought to be three major factors influencing early or premature development of arteriosclerosis. These original risk factors were elevated cholesterol, elevated blood-pressure and smoking. However, we now know that many more factors significantly influence the process. These include the following: heredity, diabetes mellitus, gender, age, obesity, sedentary lifestyle and dietary habits.

Heredity, of all these factors, is the most important. Genetic factors contribute to an individual's susceptibility or resistance to cardiovascular disease. In addition, a substantial part of the susceptibility and response to dietary factors is genetic in origin. Absolute control of the hereditary factor would involve picking our own parents, but for most of us this is not an option! Those individuals with a strong family history of arteriosclerotic cardiovascular disease should be especially aware of the other risk factors so they can alter their lifestyles to minimize the negative influence on their system.

Smoking is a factor we all have the ability to

control. The use of tobacco in all forms promotes the development of arteriosclerosis through a variety of mechanisms. The nicotine in tobacco is a powerful constrictor of blood vessels causing reduced blood flow and a greater workload on the heart. Smokers have lower levels of plasma antioxidants. We believe this makes them more susceptible to early plaque formation in arterial walls. The beneficial effects of many otherwise successful operations, such as, coronary artery bypass for complications of arteriosclerosis, are more than cut in half by patients continuing to smoke.

Diabetes mellitus has long been associated with early, diffuse and, often, prematurely fatal arteriosclerosis. However, the diabetics most severely affected are the eighty-five percent or so who are insulin resistant. These individuals require increasingly higher plasma insulin levels to achieve the same result in regulating blood glucose. Elevated plasma insulin promotes fat deposits and appears to promote smooth muscle growth in arterial walls. Both of these processes are involved in "plaque" formation. Also, high levels of insulin probably increase coagulability which obviously leads to easier clot formation and arterial occlusion.

High blood pressure, or hypertension, is classified as "essential" in over ninety percent of instances. This means we really do not know its cause, but we do know that it produces extra stress on both the heart and arterial system. The diastolic, or "bottom pressure" in the blood pressure reading, is the force or resistance the heart and blood vessels are subjected to during the relaxation phase of the cardiac cycle, or heartbeat. The greater the stress during this phase, the more accelerated the aging, or deterioration, of the arterial walls. This leads to loss of elastic tissue, cracking and, as we have seen earlier, plaque formation. Certainly, controlling blood pressure reduces stress on the cardiovascular system and promotes better long-term wear.

Hyperlipidemia (increased fat in the blood), especially hypercholesterolemia (elevated cholesterol), is associated with early arteriosclerosis. Cholesterol is a component of plaque formation. Cholesterol also is vital to the proper function of many bodily processes, such as, steroid formation and the synthesis of lipoproteins (fat and protein combinations present in the blood) which are both necessary for vital metabolic activities. Researchers also believe there is a link between cholesterol and insulin since insulin-resistant diabetics, those with high plasma levels of insulin, have abnormally elevated cholesterol levels. The predominant cholesterol component in these individuals is the LDL (low density lipid) fraction which is frequently referred to as "bad" cholesterol. Some components of cholesterol, such as, the HDL (high density lipid) fraction, especially HDL-2 and HDL-3, exert a protective effect on the cardiovascular system.

Gender is a factor in the development of arteriosclerosis, and, in this instance, women have an advantage at least until menopause. Estrogen in premenopausal women decreases blood plasma insulin levels. As we have seen in the previous chapter, this imparts a significant protective influence on the cardiovascular system as it relates to the development of arteriosclerosis. After menopause the incidence of arteriosclerosis in women begins to approach that seen in men.

Even in the absence of all risk factors, arteriosclerosis will occur; it is the natural aging process of our arteries. The theoretical maximum life expectancy of the cardiovascular system is approximately one hundred and twenty years. There is a fine line between arteriosclerosis as an aging process and as a disease. In the elderly its presence is often termed normal aging only to be reclassified as a disease when problems related to it arise. Rest assured, if we live long enough, we will develop arteriosclerosis, but consider the alternative!

Obesity has long been associated with early cardiovascular system problems. In age-adjusted populations where obesity is low, life expectancy is greater. Just compare France and the United States. Between the ages of sixteen and fifty, the French have fifty percent less obesity and twenty percent less cardiovascular and cholesterol problems than their United States counterparts. Excess body fat is deposited throughout all body tissues, and the cardiovascular system is no exception. The additional weight imposed by the extra pounds also creates an extra workload for the cardiovascular system.

A sedentary lifestyle or more aptly stated, lack of exercise, definitely does not have a positive influence on the cardiovascular system. Inactivity may not be significantly harmful, but reasonable exercise is beneficial. Exercise decreases blood pressure, decreases serum lipoproteins (especially the bad cholesterol components), decreases obesity, decreases insulin resistance, stimulates clot absorption and reduces the tendency for clot formation. Therefore, exercise positively influences many of the risk factors governing the fitness of the cardiovascular system.

"We are what we eat" is an old adage familiar to almost everyone, but today this is becoming especially more important as we better understand the full spectrum of nutrition and its effect on our various organ systems, especially the cardiovascular system. What we eat may no longer be as important as what happens to it and what metabolic effects it ultimately imparts.

Although fats and meats - especially red meats - have fallen in disfavor, and carbohydrates are definitely "in," has anyone stopped to think what happens to excess sugar which is the end product of carbohydrate metabolism? Some sugar is used in our blood to maintain an adequate circulating blood-glucose level, and some will replete glycogen stores in the liver and muscles. But what happens to the rest? It is converted to **FAT** (Guyton, 1986)! Yes, most of our body fat comes from ingested sugar, not ingested fat. This conversion is facilitated by the hormone insulin.

Additionally, insulin tends to block lipolysis, the conversion of fat back to glucose. So individuals with elevated insulin levels have a more difficult time burning fat for energy. Simply stated, they have a hard time losing weight!

Insulin plays a very important role by influencing many of the other factors we have been discussing. An increased insulin level also promotes fat deposition and growth of smooth muscle cells in the arteries (both necessary for plaque formation), and thus increases the tendency for clot formation. Two factors already discussed, estrogen and exercise, both decrease insulin resistance and are known to have a beneficial effect in retarding the arteriosclerosis process on the cardiovascular system.

However, one group of individuals, regardless of how well they positively influence most of the significant risk factors, appear to develop an early, diffuse type of arteriosclerotic cardiovascular disease which often leads to premature heart attacks, strokes and complications of hypertension. This group is comprised of insulin-resistant diabetics in whom the only primary measurable abnormality is elevated insulin levels. It has become readily apparent to us, as well as others, that insulin has many influences on the recognized processes responsible for the development of cardiovascular disease through arteriosclerosis. Therefore, the key to improving performance and health through nutrition involves insulin.

Modulating insulin secretion through diet may just be the most important variable influencing the development of cardiovascular disease. The next chapter will discuss how this modulation is accomplished as well as how it affects weight gain or loss.

X
THE DIET CONCEPT

Modulating insulin secretion is the key to our Sugar Busters'diet. Successfully controlling insulin will allow you to unlock improved performance and health through nutrition. To control insulin you must control the intake of sugar, both the refined variety and the natural sugars abundant and stimulative in carbohydrates. This is successfully achieved by selecting a nutritional or dietary concept which modulates insulin secretion in a positive fashion.

We cannot survive without insulin, but we can survive a lot better without too much insulin. Therefore, we recommend selecting foods in forms which stimulate insulin secretion in a more deliberate, controlled manner rather than those that cause the immediate outpouring of this hormone. Eating in this way will result in lower average insulin levels in our blood throughout any given period. This in turn has a markedly beneficial effect on reducing fat synthesis and storage as well as other influences we have seen insulin have on the cardiovascular system.

Since insulin is the key to our concept, carbohydrates become the cornerstone. The basic building block of all carbohydrates is sugar. Sugar absorbed from our digestive tract into our blood then stimulates insulin secretion to assist in the transport of sugar into cells as an energy source. The type of the ingested carbohydrate ultimately affects the rate of sugar absorption and, therefore, insulin secretion.

Refined sugar and processed grain products, stripped of their coatings of pulp and fiber, are almost immediately absorbed in a very concentrated fashion resulting in rapid secretion of large quantities of insulin. A diet of refined sugar and processed grain products, therefore, produces a rather marked elevation in average insulin levels throughout a twenty-four hour period. The additional insulin is then available to promote fat deposition as well as many other previously discussed undesirable effects.

However, many carbohydrates in an unrefined form, such as, whole grains require further digestive alteration before absorption. This in turn causes a proportionate reduction in the rate and quantity of insulin secretion - a modulation of insulin secretion. The end result is lower average insulin levels and less fat synthesis, storage and weight gain. The positive effects on our appearance and cardiovascular system become apparent.

Obviously, all carbohydrates are not bad but some carbohydrates, refined or pure, are not healthy for many of us. Many diets advocate eliminating almost all fat and meat, especially red meat, from our nutritional intake. Although many people do eat too much fat, some fat is necessary in our diets for the synthesis of steroids, lipopro-teins and other substances necessary for the proper metabolic operations of our bodies. But again, remember; it probably is not as much the ingested fat that makes one obese but the ingest-ed carbohydrates that are converted through the influence of insulin to fat.

Likewise, lean meats are important to our nutri-tional well-being. Not only do they supply much-needed protein, the building blocks of our bodies, but also ingested protein stimulates glucagon secretion. Glucagon, also from the pancreas, promotes the breakdown of stored fat creating a "fat loss" for our bodies.

The picture should now become clear. A diet concept based on natural sugars, such as, in fruits and low-glycemic carbohydrates, whole grains with their fiber, lean meats, and fats in moderation, biochemically modulates the insulin-glucagon relationship. This will result in overall body fat loss and a reduction of the adverse effects of insulin on our cardiovascular system.

Alcohol in reasonable amounts may theoretically be beneficial. Alcohol increases the HDL, or good cholesterol component (both HDL-2 and HDL-3), decreases plasma fibrinogen, and decreases platelet stickiness and aggregation. These actions all tend to reduce the development of arteriosclerosis and are derived from all forms of alcohol. However, red wine appears to be more beneficial than other forms of alcohol.

Grape skins, which are included in red wine's processing, contain a variety of bioflavonoids called Vitamin P which may further decrease platelet's adhesiveness or their tendency to stick to arterial walls. The bioflavonoids are more concentrated in the young red wines and precipitate out with aging.

The curve for the relationship between alcohol consumption and mortality is U-shaped and is shown in Figure 5, page 102. In moderation there is a potential benefit to our cardiovascular system, but in excess the curve changes quickly to the detriment of the consumer. Therefore, responsible use of alcohol is a must.

Contrary to public opinion, alcohol is responsible for considerably more health-related problems than even tobacco. An aspirin a day, coupled with eating grapes, can impart more safely to our bodies all the beneficial effects ascribed to alcohol consumption.

You have now completed the more technical portion of our book, and although we cannot award you with an M.D. in digestion, metabolism or cardiology, you should be equipped much better to understand the more practical suggestions on eating for good health and weight loss that follow. The conversations with your own doctors and nutritionists or dietitians also should become more interesting!

In summary, the basis of our concept is to have a positive influence on insulin and glucagon secretion through nutrition. This is achieved by eating a diet composed of natural (unrefined) sugars, whole (unprocessed) grains, fiber, lean meats, fruits, vegetables and alcohol (in moderation). Eating these foods in proper combinations also is very important and will be discussed in Chapters XI and XII.

*Deaths From Cancer, Heart Disease, Strokes & Accidents

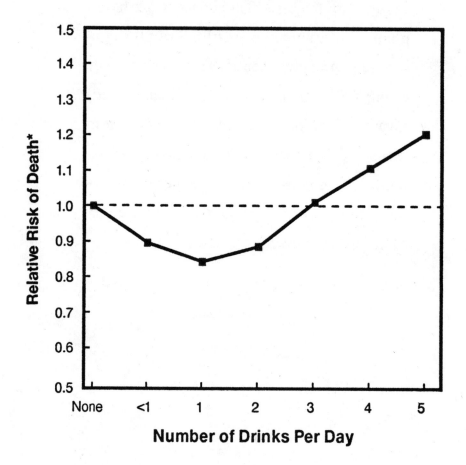

Modified from:
Marmot & Brunner, 1991

Figure 5

XI
ACCEPTABLE FOODS AND SUBSTITUTES

What foods can we really eat? Principles of metabolism and concepts of nutrition provide us with justification and guidance, but the bottom line of any diet is choosing the proper things to eat. In this chapter we hope to give you the advice and examples to make this choice easy. In addition, we will comment briefly on caffeine, artificial sweeteners and spices which are part of our everyday diet.

But first, let's look at some notable exceptions that probably will surprise you. "Potatoes are for pigs and corn for cattle;" so say the French and with good reason. They fatten these animals just as they fatten us. Potatoes, beets, carrots and many other root vegetables are simply starch, a storage form of glucose. Once inside our digestive tracts, they are converted quickly to pure sugar. Their absorption is rapid, and the resulting insulin response is very significant.

How many of us, for the sake of dieting, have not eaten a tender, juicy steak but instead have eaten a baked potato with all the fixings? If we scooped out a baked potato and filled the skin with sugar, would you eat it? Certainly not! However, that is exactly what you are doing when you eat a baked potato because it is quickly converted to sugar in your stomach.

Hybrid corn that has large, fleshy kernels causes the same large and rapid insulin response. Maize, the original Indian corn, has smaller kernels and more fiber, therefore, having a much more moderate absorption and insulin release. Many of the native American Indians became overtly diabetic when they altered their diets and started eating the modern hybrid variety of corn (Knowles, 1990). This again was the result of more than the accustomed sugar-load with its expected increased insulin response.

So to the list of refined sugar and processed grain products, especially white bread and white rice, now add potatoes, carrots, beets and corn. However, the list of recommended foods is quite extensive. Let's see what we **can** eat and enjoy (Fig. 6 & Fig. 7).

Figure 6

FOOD GROUPS

MEATS (lean)

beef*	pheasant
lamb*	partridge
pork*	elk
venison	dove
fish	duck*
shellfish	goose*
chicken*	antelope
turkey*	rabbit
quail	alligator

*trimmed or skinned

VEGETABLES

beans	squash
lentils	zucchini
peas	mushrooms
spinach	asparagus
turnip greens	artichokes
lettuce	hearts of palm
watercress	okra
cabbage	cauliflower
celery	broccoli
cucumber	brussel sprouts
dill pickles	eggplant
radishes	mirliton
bell peppers	turnips
onions	pumpkin
tomatoes	sweet potatoes

FRUIT

apples	tangerines
lemons	oranges
satsumas	limes
pears	mangos
cherries	peaches
berries	dates
pineapples	kiwis
apricots	grapes
grapefruits	plums
melons	avocados

DAIRY PRODUCTS

milk	yogurt
cheese	cream
eggs	butter

GRAINS & CEREALS

Whole-grain products (without sugar, dextrose, maltose, honey, molasses, brown sugar or corn syrup)

> whole-grain breads
> whole-grain pasta
> whole-grain rice
> shredded wheat
> wheat bran
> oat bran
> natural grains
> oatmeal

MISCELLANEOUS

nuts
spices*
garlic
chocolate (60% or greater cocoa)
Tabasco sauce
coffee**
tea**
colas with artificial sweeteners***
fruit juices without added sugar
olive oil, canola oil or peanut oil
peanut butter without added sugar
pure fruit jelly without added sugar

*   Spices are generally allowable but have little if any nutritional value.

**   Most individuals should consume no more than two to three caffeinated beverages daily. Caffeine will potentiate cardiac irregularity, high blood pressure, gastric acid secretion and appetite. Sudden cessation of caffeine may produce temporary withdrawal symptoms, such as, headache and irritability.

*** Artificial sweeteners are not harmful to the vast majority of individuals. However, they have no nutritional value.

In stores in America, it is extremely difficult to find many of these meats, vegetables or cereals (packaged or canned) without one or more of the sugar additives. Also beware of sauces, such as, ketchup and most bar-b-que sauces that are laced with one or more forms of sugar. Most commercial salad dressings contain one or more forms of sugar.

Although the glycemic indexes of the listed carbohydrates are moderate to low, someone can not expect to eat three or four portions of allowable breads, beans, sweet potatoes, etc. at a meal and not gain or retain weight! You should not consume any significant amount of allowable carbohydrates if you are consuming a high-fat meal.

Lastly, we have decided that "low-fat" on a label usually translates to "high-sugar"!

Figure 7

FOODS TO AVOID	ACCEPTABLE SUBSTITUTES
potatoes (red or white)	broiled tomatoes with cheese, sweet potatoes (yams) or mushrooms
white rice	brown rice
corn (including popcorn, cornbread and meal)	lentils, beans or okra
carrots beets	broccoli, celery, asparagus, squash, hearts of palm or artichokes
white bread	whole-grain (stone ground) breads, without added sugar, or whole-grain pasta
all refined sugar and refined white flour products, such, as, cookies, cakes, etc.	nutrasweet, fructose, sugar-free ice cream, sugar-free yogurt, sugar-free vanilla ice cream and diet root beer (float)

Having learned to make the right choices in each major food group, now we need to look at proper eating patterns and food combinations.

XII
EATING PATTERNS

All successful nutritional concepts involve the "what," "why," "when" and "how." In the preceding chapters we have discussed the "what" (low sugar) and "why" (regulate insulin secretion), but now we need to address the "when" and "how" that will bring everything together into three full meals and an occasional snack.

Multiple meals stimulate less overall insulin secretion than one or two large feedings because the frequent missing of meals will alter the body's response to insulin secretion, causing increased fat storage. Therefore, we should strive to consume three balanced meals every day.

In addition, since most cholesterol is manufactured at night when we are sleeping, a large meal of any type should not be eaten just before going to bed. Following this advice also should reduce or even eliminate most indigestion or heartburn which often awakens us in the middle of the night.

Appropriate snacks are encouraged, and most fruit, except bananas and raisins, which have a high glycemic index, is ideal for this occasion. Fruit should be eaten no closer than a half hour before or several hours after a main meal. Fruit is digested primarily in the small intestine, and when eaten with other solids, its emptying from the stomach is delayed. This allows fermentation which produces gas formation, indigestion, and often a "bloated" sensation.

Fructose, the basic sugar in fruit, stimulates less insulin secretion than glucose from other carbohydrate sources. However, when fructose is absorbed in the presence of an already elevated blood sugar, as would be the case during and immediately after a meal, its ability to stimulate insulin secretion is greatly magnified. Consequently, fruit alone as a snack is very beneficial but in combination with other foods is actually harmful. Fruit juice may be consumed prior to a meal, such as, breakfast, since fluid empties much quicker from the stomach than solids, especially if the juice is drunk first.

In general, fluids should be drunk in small quantities during meals. "Washing" food down frequently causes the bypass of proper chewing which is necessary to break food into smaller, more appropriate particles for better digestion. Excess fluid with meals also dilutes the digestive juices which reduces their ability to thoroughly interact with food not only in the mouth but also in the stomach. This may result in partially digested food entering the small intestine which can cause cramping to occur.

Fluids may be consumed at your leisure between meals. But be careful because most colas and even popular sport drinks are loaded with sugar and some also contain large quantities of caffeine. Regular coffee and tea can also present the problem of too much caffeine. We believe consumtpion of large quantities of water is good.

Alcoholic beverages present a slightly different problem. Alcohol consumed with food (full stomach) is absorbed more slowly, which causes less insulin secretion and potentially less intoxicating effects. Therefore, if you choose to consume alcohol, do so on a full stomach and only in reasonable quantities. As a word of caution, mixers for drinks usually contain a lot of sugar as does beer, so neither is considered particularly healthy. A dry (low-sugar) red wine is the preferred alcoholic beverage.

Some diets have recommended against mixing certain carbohydrates, such as, pasta and rice with protein. These combinations supposedly stimulate the secretion of competing digestive enzymes. We believe the problem is not so much the carbohydrate-protein combination but the type of carbohydrate which is consumed. For example, a meal of meat balls, without added sugar, and whole grain spaghetti is allowed. As the list in the previous chapter indicates, most unrefined or unprocessed carbohydrates are acceptable. Of course, starches in most forms (except sweet potatoes which contain a considerable amount of fiber) are harmful and should not be eaten either alone or in combination with other foods. Sorry, no meat and potatoes except for sweet potatoes!

Shoppers beware! Even the best intentions can go awry. Producers of foods have made it difficult for us to eat healthily. Most breakfast cereals, although advertised as being "the best product for your health," are laced with either white sugar, brown sugar, molasses, corn syrup or honey. In fact, it is difficult to purchase a pure natural-grain cereal. They do exist, but to find them you must read closely the fine print on the side of the box. The same problem applies to bottled, canned or other packaged foods, sauces and dressings. Almost all of them have significant amounts of added sugar. Of course, fresh vegetables are your healthiest choice, followed by those that are quick frozen and those canned or bottled without added sugars.

Whole-grain (stone ground), not "wholemeal," breads, rolls, muffins, etc. are also available in most large or specialty grocery stores. But you must be careful that our old nemesis, sugar, has not been added in one form or another. When we really begin to look at what we are eating, we quickly realize just how much sugar is present in almost everything we have been eating. To remind you where this has gotten us, refer again to Figure 2 on page 43.

As you now begin to select foods and plan your meals and snacks, remember sugar and high glycemic carbohydrates are what you need to watch. Sugar stimulates insulin secretion which instructs our bodies' metabolism to create, store and hold fat. In contrast, protein stimulates glucagon secretion which does just the opposite of insulin. Glucagon instructs our metabolism to mobilize and convert fat back to glucose which reduces our fat stores and waistlines.

A diet that reduces insulin secretion while at the same time enhances glucagon secretion is the most beneficial. This method of eating reduces body fat and cholesterol as well as the many health problems caused by both of them. Therefore, good dietary sources of protein are a must. All lean, trimmed meats, such as, beef, fish and fowl are recommended. Other excellent and healthy protein sources are eggs, cheese and nuts. Remember; it is not necessarily the fat you eat but the fat you create from sugar that is ruining your appearance and health.

You should now be getting hungry for what you really like but previously thought you should not eat. Light the grill, and let's see what's for dinner. Figure 8 contains an example of a healthy breakfast, lunch and dinner followed by an example, in Figure 9, of what most of us have historically consumed in a typical day.

Figure 8

SUGAR BUSTERS' DIET

(Balanced toward slimness and health)

Breakfast - Grapefruit, orange or apple - 1/2 hour before; shredded wheat, skim milk and Equal. Or, orange juice - 1/2 hour before; two eggs; occasionally ham, bacon or sausage; a slice of whole-grain toast (with butter); and decaf coffee or tea.

Mid-morning snack - Fruit or almonds, walnuts or pecans; or peanut butter with whole fruit jelly (both without added sugar) on rye crackers; or decaf diet drink or coffee.

Lunch - Green salad with olive oil and red wine vinegar or another sugarless dressing (even blue cheese!); full-sized portion of grilled fish or chicken with green or yellow vegetables; whole-wheat matzos, rye crisp crackers or rice cakes; decaf coffee, tea, or water. No dessert.

Mid-afternoon snack - Fruit or nuts or a high cocoa content chocolate (greater than 60% cocoa), or decaf coffee or diet cola.

Dinner - Large green salad, steak, lamb chops, veal chops, hamburger steak, etc.; green or yellow vegetables, beans, sauteed onions, mushrooms, and bell peppers (in olive oil); water; sugar-free ice cream and diet root beer (float); or just the sugar-free ice cream and sugar-free chocolate sauce with pecans; or a slice or two of cheese and a glass of wine.

Before bed - The above float, if not consumed earlier, or a handful of nuts.

This basic diet, with ample calories and fat (but low-sugar or low-glycemic carbohydrates) has allowed most of our patients to lose weight, keep it off and also lower their cholesterol by an average of 15% - all this and feeling and functioning better in the process.

Figure 9

EXAMPLE OF THE TYPICAL
"BALANCED AMERICAN DIET"

(Balanced toward fatness and disease!)

Breakfast - Orange juice with sweet rolls, granola or cereal (all laced with sugar), biscuits or toast with jelly...all bad except the juice which, when consumed with sugared or refined carbohydrates, is also bad. Caffeinated coffee or tea which, although not really bad in moderation, will stimulate insulin secretion.

Mid-morning snack - More coffee or tea (caffeinated) or a sugar-saturated cola (commonly containing about an inch and a half of liquid sugar).

Lunch - Turkey sandwich with mayonnaise (high glycemic bread plus fat and sugar in the mayonnaise) or a luncheon salad with a dressing laced with "sugar". Caffeinated tea or cola.

Mid-Afternoon - More coffee, tea or colas.

Dinner - Broiled, skinned chicken, baked potato (ugh!) with margarine, one green vegetable (yea!), rolls (hello, insulin!), fruit salad (so much for rapid stomach emptying), more iced tea or decaffeinated coffee (yea!) and probably a dessert (well, at least it tasted good!). *Before bed* - skim milk and cookies!

The above diet, while not necessarily high calorie or high fat, will not let - much less cause - you to lose weight unless you are blessed with a better than average metabolism. The person who consumed a high-glycemic diet consisting of a sandwich with white bread (processed grain), potatoes and cookies (refined sugar) had a high level of insulin in his body all day and half the night! Why are Americans and several other westernized countries' populations so obese (one in three Americans are obese) and fraught with a high incidence of diabetes? Right on! Diets of excessive sugar and high-glycemic carbohydrates "spike" the insulin.

You choose which diet makes the most sense!

XIII
CONCLUSION

In health care, transportation, telecommunications, etc., tremendous strides have been and are continuing to be made. This is not so for nutrition and dieting. Our ancestors ate better, often out of necessity, than we do today. How they ate is why our digestive system has evolved to what it is today. Sure, vitamins and other food supplements have been improved, and we constantly get to eat a variety of foods with their varying vitamins and minerals. But eating in general has caused our health to markedly deteriorate and has prevented a significant increase in life expectancy for middle-aged man. Refining and processing most of what we eat has been an unfortunate nutritional disservice, particularly the introduction of refined sugar. Our health has suffered as a result.

The evidence for this deterioration has been rather obvious for decades. The insulin dependent diabetic gained weight and his cholesterol continued to rise no matter how carefully he followed his "doctor's" instructions. Many individuals have given up meat entirely only to have their cholesterol levels increase and their vascular disease progress rapidly.

Nutritionists and dietitians "looked but did not see." Dufty and Montignac began to see. However, because they were not professionally trained in nutrition, many so-called professionals scoffed at or ridiculed them and even suggested they were charlatans.

The world of nutrition is not flat but round! Previous concepts appeared plausible, but now we have the scientific basis to prove them wrong. Most of our body fat is from ingested sugar (carbohydrates), not ingested fat. This is driven by the effects of insulin and aptly proved in the insulin-resistant diabetic. By modulating insulin secretion through diet, individuals are able to significantly influence body fat, cholesterol, diabetes and the progression of arteriosclerosis and its subsequent complications. In addition, diet can regulate glucagon secretion which has additional beneficial effects on fat metabolism.

Eating should be an enjoyable and pleasurable experience while contributing to our performance and health. Many have written about sugar and its harmful effects. We have taken this premise, verified by current and historical data, and expanded it to include our belief that *insulin* is the key. The nutritional and dietary concepts presented in *Sugar Busters!* are consistent with stimulating the ideal levels of insulin and glucagon secretions.

In addition to pleasuring our palates, the concepts proposed in *Sugar Busters!* should be good news for the cattle ranchers, sheep ranchers, hog farmers, dairy farmers and egg producers who recently have been much maligned by various health and nutrition groups. These foods are good for us today just as they were good for our distant ancestors.

With our approach, many individuals already have experienced significant weight loss and reduction in cholesterol (an average of approximately fifteen percent) as well as improvement in performance which is so vital to everyone's success. In addition, many diabetics have been successful in acheiving much better regulation of their blood sugar levels. We feel the same opportunity is available to you by following the recommendations on nutrition and diet we offer in *Sugar Busters!*

Bon Appetit!

XIV
LAYMAN'S GLOSSARY

Aminoacids - the building blocks of all protein. There are nine essential, or necessary, aminoacids which the body cannot make itself and which must be provided from the foods we eat.

Amylase - enzymes secreted by the salivary glands and the pancreas that break down carbohydrates.

Antioxidants - chemical compounds that readily accept an oxygen free radical, thus inhibiting the oxidation of polyunsaturated fatty acids which are important to maintaining cellular health. Vitamins A, C and E are antioxidants.

Atheroma - (also referred to as a plaque) is a deposit of cholesterol, calcium and platelets in the lining of major vessels eventually leading to blockage.

Arteriosclerosis - the process of hardening of arteries through the formation of plaques on the inner lining of major blood vessels.

Beta cells - specialized cells in the pancreas responsisble for the production and secretion of insulin.

Bioflavonoid - compounds found in nature mostly as yellow pigments which contain no nutritional value but which may help preserve the health of arterial walls by reducing their cholesterol content.

Blood clot - coagulated or congealed blood.

Calorie - the unit of heat (energy) required to raise 1 kilogram of water 1 degree celsius.

Carbohydrates - chemical compounds containing carbon, hydrogen and oxygen. Carbohydrates are made of sugar.

Cholesterol - a compound belonging to a family of substances called sterols. It usually combines with fat when it is circulated in the blood for distribution to cells.

Complex carbohydrate - a carbohydrate with a more complex structure, such as, starch or glycogen. The degree of complexity does not indicate necessarily the rate at which the carbohydrate is digested.

Diabetes mellitus, Type I - a disease characterized by the lack of insulin and the resulting elevated blood glucose (sugar) levels.

Diabetes mellitus, Type II - a disease characterized by resistance of the cells in the body to the actions of insulin and which also leads to elevated blood glucose (sugar) levels.

Energy - capacity to produce motion or heat.

Free fatty acid - the structural component of fat.

Fructose - a simple sugar found in fruits. Its insulin stimulating effect, while modest when consumed alone, can be magnified when consumed with other foods.

Gastric emptying - the process of emptying food from the stomach or the time required to empty a meal.

Glucagon - hormone secreted by the pancreas which helps regulate blood sugar and metabolize stored fat.

Glucose - the form in which sugar circulates in the bloodstream; the body's main energy source.

Glycemic Index - how rapidly a carbohydrate food is digested into glucose and how much it causes the blood sugar (glucose) to rise (Figure 4).

Glyceride - a group name for fats. Mono, di and triglycerides, which contain one, two or three fatty acids, are the main constituents of fats.

Glycerol - a constituent of fats. Chemically it is an alcohol which combines with fatty acids to produce fats

Glycerol-3-phosphate - a metabolic product which occurs in the transformation of glucose to triglycerides.

Glycogen - a complex form of glucose which is stored in the liver and muscle to be used to meet energy needs.

HDL cholesterol - high density lipoprotein cholesterol thought to be protective for heart disease.

High density lipoproteins (HDL) - lipoproteins carrying cholesterol from the cells to the liver for breakdown and elimination from the body, probably the single best determinant of risk for coronary artery disease and heart attacks.

Hyperglycemia - abnormally elevated blood glucose (sugar) level.

Hyperlipidemia - abnormally elevated blood lipids, usually either cholesterol or triglycerides or both.

Hypertension - persistently elevated blood pressure.

Insulin - hormone secreted by the pancreas. It lowers blood sugar by allowing the transport of glucose into the cells.

Insulin resistance - failure of insulin to exert its normal effect of allowing glucose into cells. This causes a rise in blood glucose (sugar) levels, and therefore, triggers the need for still more insulin.

LDL cholesterol - low density lipoprotein cholesterol, thought to be a major risk factor for heart disease.

Lipase - enzymes secreted by the pancreas that digest fats.

Lipid - a fat of either plant or animal origin.

Lipogenesis - the formation of fat from glucose.

Lipolysis - the conversion of stored fat to glucose.

Lipoproteins - combination of fat and proteins which circulate in the bloodstream. They function as the major carriers of lipids.

Lipoprotein lipase - a very important enzyme in the storage of fat.

Low density lipoproteins (LDL) - lipoproteins which are important in the transport of cholesterol.

Lymphatic system - vessels and lymph tissue which drain tissue fluid back into the cardiovascular system. It is the main route of absorption of fats from the small intestine.

Metabolism - the sum of all the chemical and physiological processes by which the body grows and maintains itself and by which it breaks matter down into a new state.

Modulate - regulate or control the flow of.

Monounsaturated fats - fat molecules containing only one double bond. Examples are olive oil, peanut oil and canola oil.

Obesity - the presence of excess body fat.

Pancreas - an important organ which produces both insulin and glucagon as well as digestive enzymes, such as, lipase.

Plasma fibrinogen - protein used in making blood clots.

Plaque - deposits of cholesterol, calcium and platelets on the lining of major vessels.

Platelets - elements in blood that are important in the clotting process by sticking to each other and starting the process of clot formation.

Polyunsaturated fats - fat molecules containing two or more double bonds. Most vegetable oils are polyunsaturated.

Saturated fats - fat molecules containing carbon atoms fully bound with hydrogen atoms, such as, most animal fats.

Simple sugars - also known as monosaccharides. The most important are glucose, fructose and galactose (sugar in milk).

Sterols - complex steroids, one of which is cholesterol.

Syndrome X - the combination of two or more of the following: insulin resistance, elevated insulin levels, elevated triglycerides, obesity and hypertension.

Synthesis - the manufacture or creation of a new substance.

Triglycerides - the main type of stored fat in most animal systems.

Type I diabetes mellitus - a disease characterized by the lack of insulin and the resulting elevated blood glucose (sugar) levels.

Type II diabetes mellitus - a disease characterized by resistance of the cells in the body to the actions of insulin and which also leads to elevated blood glucose (sugar) levels.

Very low density lipoproteins (VLDL) - Lipoproteins which are important in transport of fatty components.

XV
REFERENCES

Anderson, K.M., Castelli, W.P., Levy, D. Cholesterol and mortality: 30 years of follow-up from the Framingham study. JAMA 1987, 257, 2176-2180.

Artaud-Wild, S.M., Connor, S.L., Sexton, G., Connor, W.E. Differences in coronary mortality can be explained by differences in cholesterol and saturated fat intakes in 40 countries but not in France and Finland: a paradox. Circulation 1993, 88, 2771-2779.

Cardiovascular disease risk factors: new areas for research. WHO Technical Report Series 1994, 841.

deLorgeril, M., Mamelle, N., Salem, P. A mediterranean type diet in the secondary prevention of coronary heart disease. Circulation 1993, 88 (Suppl.), I-635.

Dufty, William. *Sugar Blues.* New York: Warner Books, 1976.

Guyton, Arthur C., *Textbook of Medical Physiology,* 7th Ed. Philadelphia: W.B. Saunders 1986.

Holmes, F. L. *Lavoisier and Chemistry of Life.* Madison: University of Wisconsin Press, 1985.

Jenkins DJA et. al. Glycemic index of foods: a physiological basis for carbohydrate exchange. Am J. Clin Nutr 1981, 34, 362-66.

Jenkins DJA et. al. AM J Clin Nutr 1987, 46, 968-75.

Joslin's *Diabetes Mellitus* edited by Kahn, C. Ronald and Weir, Gordon C. 1994, p. 99.

Knowles, W.C. et. al. Diabetes mellitus in the Pima Indians; incidences, risk factors and pathogenesis. Diabetes Metab Rev 1990.

Leibel, R.L., Rosenbaum, J., Hirsch, J. Changes in energy expenditure resulting from altered body weight. New England Journal of Medicine 1995, 332, 621.

Marmot, M., Brunner, E. Alcohol and cardiovascular disease: the status of the U-shaped curve. British Medical Journal 1991, 303, 565-568.

Montignac, Michel. *Dine Out & Lose Weight*. Paris: Artulen, 1991.

O'Keefe, Jr., J.J., Lavie, Jr., C.J., McCallister, B.D. Insights into the pathogenesis and prevention of coronary artery disease. Mayo Clinic Proceedings 1995, 70, 69-79.

Skrabanek, Petr, *Fat Heads*. National Review 1995, 43, 43-47.

Webb, P. American Journal of Clinical Nutrition 1980, 33.

Willis, Thomas. *Pharmaceutica Rationalis.* 1647.

Wilson, Jean D., Foster, Daniel W. Williams *Textbook of Endocrinology*, 8th Ed. Philadelphia: W.B. Saunders 1992.

Wolever T.M.S. et al. Beneficial Effect of Low-Glycemic Index Diet in Overweight NIDDM Subjects. Diabetes Care 1992, 15, 562-564.

XVI
VOLUNTARY
MAILBACK QUESTIONNAIRE

Dear Purchaser:
This book has the potential to reshape America and make her healthy again. We need help in determining the magnitude of the impact of this low-sugar diet. We know it will work but do not know to what degree it will catch on, be understood, be misunderstood or even uncover some specific dissenters (besides the affected industries). Please fill in the following blanks:

1. I lost_____pounds in_____weeks.

2. My cholesterol changed by_____%

3. I eliminated alcohol during my weight loss period. ☐ Yes ☐ No

4. I changed from hard spirits and beer to wine. ☐ Yes ☐ No

5. I don't drink alcohol! ☐

Continued on next page

6. I have had
   ☐ no indigestion
   ☐ little indigestion, or
   ☐ no change in indigestion while on this diet.

7. I would be willing to take a phone call from your representative to discuss my results and/or to get some of my own questions clarified. ☐ Yes ☐ No

8. Have you noticed a positive difference in your strength, stamina and performance in general? ☐ Yes ☐ No

9. Would you be interested in our developing for sale Sugar Busters' bread, sauces, salad dressing, cereal, suggested recipes and/or menus? ☐ Yes ☐ No
   If so, what in particular?

   _____

NAME (Please print):

_____

PHONE NUMBER:_____

Please mail to: SUGAR BUSTERS
                     P. O. Box 55808
                     Metairie, LA. 70055